Jim's Journey

The Story of a Young Man with Early On-set Alzheimer's

Gretchen L. Dausey

Edited by Karen Lee
Cover Design/Artwork by Gretchem L. Dausey
Designed by Gretchen L. Dausey

Order this book online at www.trafford.com
or email orders@trafford.com

Most Trafford titles are also available at major online book retailers.

Printed in Victoria, BC, Canada.

ISBN: 978-1-4251-3765-6 (soft)
ISBN: 978-1-4251-3766-3 (ebook)

*Our mission is to efficiently provide the world's finest, most comprehensive book publishing
service, enabling every author to experience success. To find out how to publish your book, your
way, and have it available worldwide, visit us online at www.trafford.com*

Trafford rev. 2/18/2010

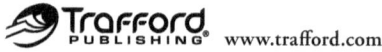 www.trafford.com

North America & international
toll-free: 1 888 232 4444 (USA & Canada)
phone: 250 383 6864 ✦ fax: 812 355 4082

I want to especially acknowledge that my sister, Karen, was very instrumental in the writing of Jim's Journey. There were countless edits and a lot of gab sessions and time spent together in getting this book into print. She was the one that I bounced a lot of ideas around and her insight with words and phrases was phenomenal.

Karen, thank you, from the bottom of my heart.

Love, Gretchen

Acceptance

You have Alzheimer's disease
And you're losing the power,
To remember- to reason - to understand
To do the simple tasks we take for granted
to put on a shoe -to button a shirt -
to read a book -to remember a face or name
It's a hard thing to understand -To accept…
Perhaps it's been the hardest for me,
For I've lived with you -
But I know - you can't help it –
Can't act otherwise…
I must take you as you are and expect - not more -But less
as the disease continues to progress.
Maude S. Newton

Used by permission of her son

W. Frank Newton

INTRODUCTION

This story needs to be told, not only for me as personal therapy and as way of putting all my thoughts in order, but to help other loved ones and caregivers have a first hand account of how Alzheimer's affects a husband and wife who have shared a life together since they were 15 and 16 and how very difficult it is in handling this dreaded disease.

There is a lot of information from doctors and the Alzheimer's Association but I couldn't find any from a personal perspective. There are many message boards on the internet that have been very helpful to me. Each entry targets a certain problem, but sometimes it is very hard to weed through it all and find what is needed.

Over the last few months, other loved ones have been coming to me asking me questions about how I have handled some of the problems that come with Alzheimer's Disease and helping Jim, my husband, get through them.

I want Jim's Journey to be able to help someone if told in whole from beginning, but as of right now there is no ending. That day will come some time in the future.

Even though this is Jim's Journey, I'm making it with him, so here's a little about me and how I came to write this.

When I was 18 months, in 1949, my Mom contracted Polio. At that time my family lived with my grandparents from both sides including an aunt and uncle off and on over several years.

Even at a young age I had learned of the limitations that my mom encountered. All through the years I watched out for my mom, of course my dad was there, but I helped out more with chores than most kids would. (At least I believe I did). My mom always told me that once the work was done that I could play. To this day I still follow that rule.

In my senior year at high school my mom fell and broke her good leg. Her left side was still left somewhat paralyzed from the polio, making it difficult for her to get around. Although she tried not to let it get in the way and not make a big deal about it, we watched out for her but sometimes there were falls. I took care of the family for awhile until she could get back on her feet. I would get the younger kids off to school before I left for school myself. Then when I would get home I would clean whatever Mom wanted and cook most of dinner. My Dad would also get things going; we worked together on keeping the house in order.

I believe this was the start of my care giving

I helped my Mom the best I could through out my life but especially when my Dad developed cancer. My Mom could not drive so I took time from work and would take him for his chemotherapy and to all his doctor visits until he passed on. I then became a part time care giver for my Mom along with the help of my sister. My Mom was a very independent lady and we tried to keep her that way even though she could only get around with a motorized scooter.

After my Dad died, my Mom stayed in her own home. She was given the opportunity to live with my brother and his wife in North Carolina, but she was adamant about her independence and remained that way until the day she died.

My Mom put all of my upbringing into focus for me when she gave me a birthday card she had made on the computer. I keep it to this day to remind me how she felt.

The front of the card has several pictures of different pairs of shoes; overlaid on it are the words "No one can fill your shoes". The inside of the card is a page titled "Love Notes" and around the the edge of the page are little red hearts.

It reads:

Born on Thursday the doctor called Grampa Kalbaugh, didn't know that your Dad was already at the hospital.

We wanted a German name for you and came up with Gretchen. Aunt Ger thought you were named after her, so you were addressed as "little Gretch" and she as "Big Gretch".

She loved it. She brought an orchid for me at the hospital and pinned it to my pillow. It was my first orchid.

Remember how you loved high heels? Gramma Kalbaugh sent them to New York. We were on our way to dance class in Schenectady and left them on the bus but we did get them back. (That is why I picked this card).

And what a great daughter you are. You had so many people influencing you as you grew and I think you got the best from each person.

Aunt Mabel, you are so like her with all your kindness, Gramma Cash who had you for six months to take care of. Gramma Gerding helped out too and of course Grammas Kalbaugh and Stewart. That is a lot for one little girl.

A lot of people helped form your personality and how great you turned out. You have truly been a blessing in Dad's and my life.

She signed it, "I love you. Happy Birthday. Mom".

In spite of all my Mom has told me of the compassion that I have, I am still in awe of the way people have come to me and wanted me to listen, to ask questions, to help. My hope is that in some small way I can help and let them know they are not alone and that others, millions of others are having the same journey.

I am 59 but I still feel like a kid inside and never in my wildest dreams would I have thought that I would come to this type of role in my life. I only tell this part of my life so that you can understand how amazed I feel of my care giving situation and know that I do this out of love.

2000

Jim's symptoms really started showing their face in 2000; at least that is when I realized something was going wrong. In hindsight I think that it may have started sooner. Doctors had said that Jim's Mom had AD, but that was only a month before she died. In later years, after Jim and I were married, Jim's mom developed cancer. She needed 24 hour care. We all did what we could, there were 3 other brothers with wives and a niece who helped out, but it just did not work. We had to put Jim's mom in a nursing home.

I don't really know if the doctors had sufficient time to test her. She was on so many medications that also could have been the cause. Two of Jim's aunts, his Mom's sisters had AD and had passed away. I keenly was aware of all these facts and of what may lie ahead for Jim.

Jim was a surveyor and field inspector for an engineering company. He had worked for them for 30 years. Jobs started moving farther north because the company was in sanitary sewers.

We live about 15 miles south of Pittsburgh, Pa. and the company wanted him to work on a project in Titusville, Pa. which is 114 miles north of Pittsburgh.

The company was not going to compensate fairly for the travel, overtime or the fact that he might stay over night at some point. No provisions were going to be made for any motel stay.

The idea Jim gave to me was that 4 or 5 of the guys would rent a house and divide the cost – again no compensation was coming from the company. Also part of the problem with this situation was Jim had never really spent any time away from me. There were a few trips the guys took on the bikes but only for a day, but being away from home added to all the frustrations.

Jim and I sat down and went over all our options and decided that if we used his 401k money to pay all the bills, we could live on my salary with out any problems.

Jim handed in his notice. I thought everything would be fine. At his retirement party some of the guys he worked with told me Jim had seemed so confused on the job site - where he was, what he was doing. They believed he had gotten lost many times.

Jim was working in Greensburg, Pa. right before he quit his job. He knew Greensburg like the back of his hand. He was running between three job sites almost everyday. When the guys told me their thoughts at the party, I put it up to stress because the company wanted Jim to work farther and farther north and be away from home.

A few weeks or so after he quit working, I got a few phone calls from the project engineer. The foreman of the construction company that Jim was supposed to be overseeing said that Jim hadn't been on the job a lot of the time. Jim was mad, saying he was there everyday.

Jim would take a walk at lunch time, he was always big on exercise, I think that after his walks he would forget that he was to return to the job site and come home instead. There were times that he would call me and tell me he was home. I didn't think much of it, because he was often home early, but after the phone calls I began to wonder.

Now that Jim was home all day, by himself, he asked me what kind of chores he should do. All I asked of him was to make sure the laundry was done, and if he wanted, to make supper once in a while. He used to make a pretty good pot of spaghetti sauce, pasta fagiole, and chili. (He had his Mom's recipes)

You have to understand something, we didn't have any children, so Jim was very spoiled and I gave him whatever he wanted. I did not want to force him to do something he didn't want to. At the time he still rode his motorcycle and I wanted him to have fun. He did take care of things rather well for awhile. As the year went on, I started noticing that he slowly quit doing things. But it didn't really register until much later.

The rest of the summer of 2000 seemed to go pretty good. I think in part because we had a lot of remodeling done and there were construction workers around the house. We had it re-sided and a new deck put on. Jim enjoyed being outside and watching all that went on. He loved being the sidewalk supervisor. There were things that didn't add up, and sometimes I really wasn't sure what was happening. But I thought he was just getting adjusted to being home by himself and not working.

2001

The changes were very subtle. Jim was repeating himself, more than I thought was normal, but being with him day in and day out; I couldn't always see the changes or be able to put two and two together.

We were avid NASCAR fans and went to Dover Downs twice a year from 1988 to 2001. We always took a long week-end and stayed in Dewey Beach. We had friends that lived in Viola, Delaware, where we would meet up with all and then off to the races. We always had enjoyable trips.

Well, in Feb. of 2001, we had the chance to go to the Daytona 500 and had over a week for vacation. Jim drove on the trip down and as I recall the drive was uneventful. There may have been a little confusion here and there, even though we had done that drive before for "Bike Week" about three times it still was somewhat unfamiliar.

Our stay at the motel was on a whole going pretty well. Jim did have a few outbursts, but there wasn't any reason or explanation for them. He seemed to be afraid of the height. We had a room up fairly high and overlooking the ocean, but he was always standing back and didn't want to be on the balcony. There were a few times when he was taking a shower and carrying on about something. I was going into the hall to get some things and his voice just vibrated through the wall. I would go back and try to calm him down before going back out again.

It was the day of the Cup race, Feb 18, 2001 (the day Dale Earnhardt Sr. died). We got to our seats okay, got situated, and then went to the refreshment stand. I got the food, Jim went to the restroom. He said he would meet me back at the seats. I thought it would be okay. He took longer than I felt he should so I kept a keen lookout for him, mentally ringing my hands. Finally I saw him, but he was in the wrong section. He had never lost his way before at any of the other races and I was nervous.

With the help of some of the people around us, I got his attention. I think he was embarrassed by them calling out his name because he never left his seat until after the race was over.

But during the race we were trying to put on our ponchos. No matter how he tried he could not figure out how to get it on. I tried to help but he kept slapping my hand away and getting really upset. Finally I just stopped trying. The rest of the race we did not say much to each other.

At this point I knew that things were very wrong and that I had to do something about it. I didn't know how I was going to do it, but I knew I had to.

It was June 2001, and it would be the last race we would ever go to. We were at the Dover race. Jim kept repeating himself, asking questions about things he should have known the answer. One of our friends asked if we had been to the Saturday race. Jim looked at me with a question on his face and told the friend no. But we had been to that race! Jim could not remember. Our friends noticed the difference in Jim, and asked me about it. This just emphasized the fact I needed to get help for Jim.

On our way home from Dover, we had to cross the bridge over the Chesapeake Bay, a rather high bridge coming from Kent Island toward Annapolis in Maryland. Jim was driving on the bridge when all suddenly he said "talk to me". Well when someone says that to you, you can never think of anything to say. Within a few seconds which sure seemed a lot longer, I was able to come up with something other than "the bridge sure is high". Finally we were off the bridge and Jim pulled over to the side. He said he had no idea what had happen to him or why, but he was quite upset and asked if I would drive the rest of the way home.

After this incident Jim told me that maybe traveling wasn't such a good idea anymore. I agreed and that was our last vacation.

During the rest of 2001 there was a lot of misunderstanding, confusion and probably quite a few arguments. I knew I had to get him to the doctors for testing; I really wasn't sure how to do this. I had spoiled Jim so much, never forcing him to do anything he didn't want to do. So how was I going to tell him that he needed to be tested for Alzheimer's??

Jim started keeping a journal of each day's events. He began on November 12, 2001 and kept it up until February 7, 2005. He kept pretty good detail of the days events. Most of the entries written were of the weather and taking his medicine. He has high blood pressure and high cholesterol, so naturally he didn't want to forget his medicine. At the time he was writing, or I should say printing, I never really looked at the journals. He seemed to be very private about them. Once in awhile, when he was busy doing something else I would take a quick peek. Later, I started reading his journals to get a better insight of his journey to help me write about it.

Jim already had an appointment scheduled for the 29th of November 2001. At this time some things were in question about the stories he would tell me about his walks in the park. I didn't really know if they were true.

Jim would walk anywhere for 5 to 7 miles a day. He would tell me it was a way of passing time until I got home from work.

Jim told one story that put the icing on the cake the morning he had his doctor's appointment. I was getting ready to go to work and he was getting ready to go to the doctors. Jim told me he was sorry about last night. He said when he was out having a few beers with his friends, they would not let him come home and that he thought he had taken two sets of his medicine.

At that point I told Jim he had been with me all night and had never gone out. As far as the medicine I told him I would call the doctor before he got there and the doctor could check him out.

I did call the doctor but I also relayed the story Jim told me of being out the night before. It was shortly after that the doctor had me make an appointment with a neurologist.

2002

Jim's journal notes stopped between February 11, 2002 and April 14, 2002. This is the time he was first diagnosed with Alzheimer's Disease. I don't know exactly the date, but it was some time in the end of February. There was a battery of blood tests and brain scans by the neurologist.

There was a visit with a psychiatrist who gave Jim about a three hour examination. At first the psychiatrist had me with them for about fifteen minutes or so and then I left so they could talk. It was shortly after that Jim had the follow up visit with the neurologist and the doctor confirmed that all the testing pointed to AD. Jim was only 55. Actually it was a month before he turned 55.

Aricept was prescribed. Jim was upset about all the events. I did try to calm his fears as best I could. I never told him that it would eventually lead to death. Maybe I was in denial.

It was at this time Jim decided to be more serious about keeping a daily journal. I got him about a dozen steno pads and he was quite happy with them.

Almost everyday up until early 2005, when he no longer kept his journal, he noted what ever the weather was to be. He had the temperatures and the conditions written done.

During car racing season, be it NASCAR, CART, INDY CARS or FORMULA I, he tried to keep track of all the events that were on TV. The times and stations were all listed. I can't tell you how many times he asked me what stations each were on. It was always the same questions. Jim would write down the numbers for the stations. As I looked over the journals those numbers were repeated over and over. Not just on one page, but all over the pages and the covers of his journal.

He had me print out all the schedules for each race venue and kept them handy for reference. He said he didn't want to miss any races, but usually what happened was Jim forgot what he was watching and would move on to some other show. Many times when a commercial would come on he would ask "what are we watching here?" When it came to TV shows the attention span was very short. He also had trouble with the remote control. You know how men are with the remote, but after awhile Jim turned it over to me. He couldn't figure out which buttons to push.

Jim would note in his journal that he was going for a walk on any given day, what time he left and came home, how many miles he walked. He would try to keep track of times for his medicine, but as I read his journal I see that he would forget and then double them up in the afternoon. The reoccurring theme was always weather and walking.

There are plenty of stories he relayed in his journal. Some were disturbing and some were humorous and some were very loving. There are some of these stories that need to be told. As I read them I feel that a lot of the notes he made allowed him to communicate much better than if he would tell them out loud. Most of the time when he had a conversation with some one it was more exaggerated than most. I know men have a way of telling tales that are a little bit more than exaggerated but some of the things that Jim would say were pretty much way out. In his writing he didn't over tell and make things bigger than they really were. I could also see that he had a lot of erasures and started over again. There is no way of telling what the original entry was.

One story was about a couple of walkers that would hassle him. One walker accused him of denting his car at the parking lot. Jim told the walker that it could not have been him and that if it was he would have had damage on his own car and there were not marks. Also Jim states in his journal that these walkers had pieces of galvanized pipe with them. Jim gave me no further explanation of the pipe. He only told me of this maybe a day or two after this confrontation happened. When he finally did tell me I said maybe it was just a bad dream.

There were many stories like this. I was getting more concerned as to how to handle this.

Jim would tell me a lot about what happened on his walks. These tales were the most disturbing to me. He told me of some kids that would taunt him with metal objects. Jim told me they were explosives and the kids would throw them at him. Jim seemed to go into some real detail about how they followed him. The way Jim told the story, the kids were always in the woods in the park, and it seemed that they always kept their distance. Jim told me of this incident happening more than once.

One of most worrisome of the tales was the one Jim told me about two brothers he met up with and would walk with him for a while. Then Jim would go in another direction to get off by himself. These two brothers would argue with each other. Jim told me the way they would talk, that he thought they either own a motel or a nursing home. Jim said that he would go at different times to try to miss them for their walk, but most of the time they would be there when Jim was. All the different things these brothers said had to do with bedding, sheets and something about oxygen. Jim sometimes didn't always say the same thing but there were always the same references. Jim described the cowboy hat the one would wear and the kind of car the other had. Jim always had the feeling that they were rich. One day Jim said that their sister had won the lottery for a lot of money. Of course I was very skeptical of these conversations, mostly because of the other stories that I felt sure were not totally true. I listened to all the tales Jim had but I wasn't sure what to believe.

Then one day Jim called me at work and said he had seen the face of the one brother on the television. Jim thought that something bad had happened but he didn't know exactly. At this point when Jim would watch TV he didn't always understand what anyone was saying. Anyway, I listened to Jim's account of what he thought he heard. After talking to him I saw this story in the paper. It had the guy's picture and a description of his car. It said his mother was ill and he was the caregiver.

The guy either forgot or didn't give his mother oxygen that day, so when she died, the guy went to some remote area and killed himself. It also mentioned that the sister had won a big lottery prize and that there was a lot of in fighting between the siblings.

It also detailed the kind of car this guy drove. Everything that was in the paper was exactly just as Jim had told me. The only thing that he couldn't tell by the way these two brothers talked was whether they had a nursing home or a motel, but from the news paper article I could understand why Jim misunderstood. So, here I was with proof that one of his bizarre stores was true, so now I wasn't sure what to believe when Jim told me his tales of his walks in the park. I did not want to pass judgment or argue about any of them. I tried only to give advice, gently of course, on what he should do. For a while he did not walk in the park. He seemed to give it some time for all of this in the news about these brothers to die down.

Most of the entries in Jim's journal were repetitious stating the time he got up or I got up. Times were marked down at to when he took his walks or when he took his medicine. Sometimes he would mark how long it took him to do something. I would look over his journal once in a while and see how long it did take and the times seemed to be too long for what it should have. He referred to the fact that it took him 40 minutes to drive the round trip to the park. We are only about 5 miles away and I don't think that would take 20 minutes to only drive one way. So it is hard to tell. Maybe he had gotten lost as he was driving.

He would remind himself to do things such as take a shower or brush his teeth. He would tell himself to work on the garage clock, but then he noted that he couldn't do it. He wanted to be able to do a lot of things but now it was starting to be difficult to coordinate his hands and he would get all mixed up. Even to put a switch plate on the wall he wasn't able to get the screw and the screw driver to work.

As more of these kind of things started to happen when there was something that needed to be done, we would call a handy man to do them. To ease over this situation and the frustration of him not being able to handle these chores, we referred to it as "let the professional do it". This made it a lot easier for Jim, so he didn't feel embarrassed.

Jim would have little funny things in his journal, too. He would put symbols next to the days that were holidays. He had "HO HO" beside Christmas, or had a pumpkin drawn beside Halloween.

On some of his comments he would use yoi or double yoi when he wasn't sure of things he wanted to do or would have to do, maybe they were things he just didn't want to do. Jim was mimicking Myron Cope, the famous Pittsburgh Steelers broadcaster.

He had loving notes in his journal too. Of course they made me cry, especially the entries on our anniversary and on my birthday. There were hearts with the arrow through them and one was outlined in green on one particular birthday of mine.

We were to go to the doctors one day and he put in his journal, "we leave for doctor appoint. with Gretchen @ my side". Next to it is a heart.

Jim would call me at work so many times that I finally got him to call me on my cell phone. I didn't have a direct line and he would get so frustrated that I was not on the phone right away. He would yell at me for not answering. Everyone where I worked knew Jim had Alzheimer's Disease. They were very understanding and knew when my cell phone rang that more than likely Jim had a problem and I needed to take the call. One particular call was about the budget and check writing. Jim told me he had been working on it for more than two hours but he got nothing done. He was worried about it. I tried to ease over it and told him I would help him when I got home. Shortly after that I started taking care of the budget and the bills.

Other incidents that happened were that he seemed to have confrontations with different people. There was one in particular that I had to intervene. Jim always seemed to smell smoke. We did the rounds on this one for a long time. Most of our neighbors have fire places or chimineas. One neighbor across the way was burning something that did smell awful. Jim marched himself over to that neighbor and confronted him. I could hear Jim's voice but couldn't really make out what was being said. Jim called the cops and went back and forth with them. Finally the police said there was nothing they could do. To try to appease Jim and seem like I would take care of it, I went to a lawyer to see what could be done. At the time I felt there was nothing, which in so many words is what the lawyer told me. But it did give me some ideas how to settle Jim down in that situation.

At one point in time Jim said our next door neighbor was burning in his fire place. He told me that there was brown smoke pouring out of the side of the house. Without really knowing what to do I asked Jim to show me. He took me out side over to the neighbor where the brick is for the chimney and put both hands on the bricks and swore there was smoke coming out of it the other day. All of a sudden Jim said "Let's get out of here". I think at that moment he came to realize that nothing was going on. The only thing I can figure was that he saw vapors from their dryer which vents out that side of their house.

I had problems many times about explaining the smoke smell. Some times I would tell him it was his shirt from being at the bar. I got him to change his shirt and then he was okay. Other times something that simple did not work. Finally I bought some of those Ionci Breeze towers from Sharper Image. Then that settled down.

2003

Going into 2003 Jim was getting much more confused. He called me at work so many times that we went way over our minutes on the cell phone. Jim would call me about everything and anything. He could never find things at home. I think I had almost everything memorized on where to find them. Then if he had misplaced what he was looking for he would have such a temper tantrum. He had a pretty bad temper when he was younger, but as he aged he seemed to mellow, but now it was starting to come back. He would get mad and hang up on me. I had to be very careful of what I said to him and how I said it. A lot of times I would call Jim back to smooth things over but usually he had half forgotten why he was mad or even what he was looking for. It was during this time that I knew I needed to be home with him. I had to be there to make sure he was okay.

Jim slowly stopped doing any more chores, which were few. He could no longer do the laundry. This is what many of the phone calls were about. He was always asking where the soap was or asked how to sort the clothes. We had to start doing the wash together on the weekends. I would try to let him think he was doing most of the work, try to let him help, but I really was doing it all. I had to start taking the clothes downstairs myself. He would trip or fall trying to go down the steps. I had to be careful that he didn't hurt himself.

Jim also enjoyed making dinner if it were some kind of a sauce dish. He used to make a mean pot of spaghetti sauce. His chili was always really good and he liked to make pasta fagioli. Jim had all his mother's recipes which were handed down from her mother. All Italian you know. There are many pictures of Jim with a big smile on his face in the kitchen stirring the sauce. I just love seeing those pictures. He always looked so happy in them.

One night Jim made a pot of sauce. He said that something was missing - it didn't taste exactly right. He told me that he must have forgotten some spices. I appeased him and said it tasted just fine, but of course there was something missing. Another night when he made chili Jim said the same thing about it. Something was missing. Again I appeased him.

Little by little he quit making dinner. He would call and ask about getting the ground meat out of the freezer and he would make dinner. When I did get home from work the meat was thawed out but that was all. Jim would move on trying to do other things and most likely forgot about the meat.

When I would get home from work I could see that he had attempted to work around the house or try to do something on the computer. There were always half way done projects that he either couldn't do or forgot he was doing them. I would go around and check what needed picked up or finished before getting dinner ready.

Jim did realize how much more I was doing at home after work and would tell me. He would say he was sorry but he couldn't always remember what had gone on during the day. A majority of his journal entries did not detail that kind of thing. Most of the entries were very short about taking his medicine and the time he left and came home from his walks.

During this period I was also part time care giver for my Mom. After my Dad passed away, I was more or less on call for her. I would go to her house on Tuesdays to take out the garbage for pickup, check to make sure she was alright and sometimes stop on the way to get her a take out order for dinner.

Jim and I would go grocery shopping for my Mom on Saturdays, spend some time with her and have dinner. On holidays I would cook over at my Mom's, go over early to get the ham or turkey in the oven. Sometimes Jim would come with me early in the day; sometimes he wanted to walk and would come over later. It worked out most of the time.

Still there was the usual mother-in-law, son-in-law relationship. Jim would grumble about it, but there were misunderstandings. Jim didn't always understand conversations, maybe he was bored and really did not listen, I am not sure. There were many times after we had gotten home that I tried to make him understand whatever the situation was and smooth ruffled feathers. Some of Jim's reasoning powers were starting to fail him. Even though there were some tense moments, not too severe, Jim was very compassionate with the fact that my Mom could not get out to do the things she wanted to and depended on us to do a lot for her.

It was in the mist of all of this that I found that I couldn't do all of these things and hold down a full time job. I already knew I need to be home to make sure Jim was okay, but now I needed to do something about it.

I had been keeping track of my pension. With all the calculations I decided I could retire at the end of 2004. This decision came in the summer of 2003, before my Mom died. I could get my lump sum payment, roll it over into an IRA and be pretty comfortable, not rich, but comfortable. I set the date of retirement for November 30, 2004. This was also our wedding anniversary date. Jim was ecstatic, he was so happy that is all he could talk about and wrote about a lot in his journal. I could turn my attention to Jim and my Mom.

Before my Mom passed away in December of 2003, there were many trips to the doctors and a few to the hospital emergency room. A few times on my way home from work, I would get a call from my Mom that she needed to get to the ER. She would call the ambulance and I would meet her at the hospital. Of course I had to call Jim, let him know what was going on and that I would be late getting home. He always told me to be careful and call him when I knew how Mom was doing. At these times Jim was very concerned and understood that my Mom needed me. He never gave me a bad time about my Mom when she had hospital stays. My sister was always there too. Together we did the best we could for my Mom.

Jim seemed to handle my Mom's funeral rather well. At this point in time he was aware of some of his difficulties and prompted him to think about himself.

My Mom and Dad were both cremated and Jim made sure to tell me he did not want that. He wanted to have a church service and be buried in a nice place. Jim really didn't say that in so many words, but I knew what he was trying to say. I told him he would have exactly what he wanted. One particular outing I knew where I thought he would like to be buried. We rode past the cemetery that was sort of out in the country, rather sunny place. Jim sort of looked it over as we passed it and agreed, but also said that he didn't want to talk about it anymore. That was enough. I agreed and kept it in the back of my mind for when the time comes.

At my Mom's funeral, family members were noticing Jim's progression into this disease. I talked to them about it. They wanted to know how he was doing. They all knew. Jim told them at the family picnic the summer before my Mom passed. We had the picnic at my Mom's house, so we didn't have to haul everything to the park. It was easier on all. However it happened to come about, the family was sitting in the living room. The way my Mom's place was set up, Jim was at the one end and everyone else was in a semi-circle at the other end. It was not very far apart, and on the intimate side.

I guess because the way every one was placed around the room, Jim had the courage to tell them all that he had Alzheimer's. The family was very quiet the whole time Jim was talking. Jim told them as much as he could about the disease, and that he was on medicine that would help him. I can't remember all that Jim had said. I sort of sat off to the side trying not to cry. I knew what was in store. Jim talked for about 15 to 20 minutes. Afterwards I could tell the family was impressed by him being open about the Alzheimer's. There were a lot of hugs and kisses. Once Jim was done talking he said it was all okay and now was time to get on with the picnic and eat.

My Mom's passing left a very big hole in my life. I do not regret any thing, I know that I did the best I could for her at the time it needed to be done. Now I needed to turn my full attention to caring for Jim.

2004

As we started into 2004 the confusion level was escalating even more. The phone calls were too numerous to count. There were so many things that needed to be done. My Mom's home had to be totally cleaned out to get ready to sell. It wasn't easy. Jim did the best he could and we had help from my sister and my brothers and their wives. A lot of Mom's things went to Goodwill. She wore a very small size and none of us girls could fit into them. All the keepsakes, jewelry, pictures and all kinds of mementos that her and my Dad had collected over 52 years of marriage was carefully divided among us all. It was a trying time. It took six months to finally sell the home, but we did okay with that.

The next milestone was Jim had to have neck surgery. He had two deteriorating discs. Once we saw the x-rays we knew why he had pain and so much discomfort. He was nervous but the doctor was a very good surgeon and had a wonderful bedside manner. That put Jim at ease. He did rather well and had a very good recovery. There were plenty of drugs so there was not much pain. This all happened in February. The day he came home from the hospital was my birthday. Needless to say there wasn't much of a celebration. But I didn't mind as long as Jim was okay and feeling much better. As I look back in hindsight, I will always wonder if this surgery could have started more of a decline in Jim. There is some discussion of sorts that leads me to believe that. He was on drugs for the pain plus the AD drugs and also for high blood pressure and cholesterol. With all that was happening to Jim, his abilities to do things were really going down hill. There were good and bad days but the bad days were starting to get more and more frequent.

It seemed no matter what I said it was always wrong or at the most inopportune time; a lot of arguments, yelling and fighting. At this point in time I did not know how to handle any of the situations that would come up. Jim's reasoning powers were on the down swing. At first not very obvious but as time went on I had to do some research on AD to know how to handle these things.

One incident that occurred, just to show that some of Jim's actions were going awry, was when we bought a snow blower. Jim no longer wanted to shovel snow. When Jim tried to use the blower, he had no clue as to how to even start it. He had been an airplane mechanic in the service and as far back as I can remember Jim always took care of the cars and always did his own work on the motorcycles.

I had gone to the store where we bought the snow blower and had the salesman show me exactly how to start it. I put numbers on each part that had to do with starting it. Jim never was able to start the snow blower. I had to do it. We only used it maybe three times.   When Jim did use it he could never drive it in a straight line. Jim ended up shoveling the snow by hand and even then it was never in a straight line. Eventually I sold the snow blower. We now have some one come and plow the snow for us when needed.

There were a few occasions over the transition period between winter and spring and over the summer months when the windows were open. Jim was very conscious of smells. The smells bothered him at different times. Jim would actually get angry about the odors, tell me to close the windows, then in only a matter of minutes he would yell at me for closing them saying it was too hot. I would try to explain, try to reason with him, but it was not working. We would go round and round on this. He just couldn't understand. The reasoning powers were literally going out the window and I was having a hard time coping with all of this. I still hadn't figured it out yet. It took me awhile to know how to ease over all of these incidents and kind of know what to say, but it took me a long time to come up with other things to say to him.

One night after dinner we were sitting in the living room. Jim was talking a blue streak covering just about every subject you could think of. He did this quite often for a few months and then all of a sudden it went away. This particular time, in the middle of the conversation, he did a complete u-turn. Jim went into a rage. He called me every name in the book, came after me swinging and hit me a couple of times.

Luckily they were not hard hits, but still he did hit me. I ran into the bedroom and cried my eyes out. Jim just did not let up in his tirade. He kept calling me names and yelling at me to get out of the house. I don't know how long it lasted but it finally stopped. A little later after Jim had calmed down, he came to me and apologized and said he was sorry. There were other times when he tried to hit me. This stage of AD thankfully did not last long. One other time he accused me of hitting him. I was only defending myself but I think he took that as me hitting him. Jim said his face was swollen and hurting. At this point I called Jim's brother for help. I explained what was going on and how I needed him to help break Jim's mood by intervening. Jim's brother and his wife were here in a matter of minutes. It took Jim a while to calm down but that action made a big difference. Jim's brother stayed for the evening and somewhere in there Jim did apologize. Once that had happen Jim's brother knew it was safe for him to go home. I am sure that particular incident would have escalated had his brother not come to the house.

One day Jim must have been frustrated that he could not get his shoes on. He threw the shoe against the wall and then hit the wall with his hand. Jim had said his hand hurt and blamed me for hitting him. This happen some time after his brother had been over. I took the bull by the horns, hoping I could nip this in the bud before it got out of hand. I put my hand on Jim's shoulder and looked him directly in the eye. Point blankly I told him in no uncertain terms, "You get this straight here and now, I did not hit you and I will never hit you. Don't ever forget that." I didn't yell, but I was very firm and aggressive in my tone. After that the hitting stopped.

There was a reoccurring theme that happened after all of these arguments and fights, Jim would fall asleep; sometimes for a few hours and sometimes for the rest of the evening. When he would wake up Jim never remembered any of it. In a way it was a relief, since I didn't have to try to explain or re-live it. It was very disturbing though knowing that Jim was forgetting. These were not little things. As far as I was concerned they were huge things that most couples would have been agonizing about for a long time.

Sound bothered Jim an awful lot. If I would rustle the newspaper too much or if the sounds came from outside he would get upset. When he heard sounds of cars going up and down the street or a dog barking, Jim would often go out to yell at what ever was making the noise. I even had to turn the ringers off on the phones. He would just get so upset. "Why were the phones ringing? Who would be calling?" I would check the answering machine to see if any one called. If someone did I would turn the answering machine down really low so he couldn't hear it to make sure the call wasn't too important and see who called. Again I would try to explain but Jim's reasoning powers were getting worse.

Finally retirement day came. Don't get me wrong, I really enjoyed my work I had been there 39 years, but is was such a relief to know I could be home with Jim now.

Little did I know what was in store for either of us.

New challenges showed their faces now that I was home 24/7 with Jim. It was only him and me. For the first time in our lives Jim had my full attention. I could really take care of him now.

2005

I started taking over the driving almost immediately after I quit working. The times that I had let Jim drive and saw how he drove and reacted to the different situations that are involved with driving, I could not in good conscience let him drive anymore. When we went anywhere, as we were going out the door I politely told him I would drive. When he put up a fuss I just told him that he chauffeured me around the first 35 years we were married; now it was my turn to chauffeur him around for the next 35 years. It took some time for me to convince Jim that I should do the driving. I would calmly tell him that he would feel terrible if there was an accident and some one got hurt, or that we may also be hurt. I told him we needed to be safe for everyone. Believe me, this was not easy and it took quite awhile, repeating and repeating until finally Jim stopped fighting me about not letting him drive. Once that was settled our outings became easier to bear.

Jim stopped walking daily. He wanted to spend all of his time with me. The first several months were a time for us to get use to being together all day long. Jim wanted to be out doing something. We would get up early. In the summer months we would be out on the porch. Jim would have coffee ready and watch the birds and the clouds. We have a great view out the back of the house. There are a lot of woods across the way and a big field. We could watch the animals, especially the wild turkeys. But he wanted to be on the go. So out we went to do many things, most anything just so he wasn't in the house. We would go for breakfast a lot and then do some shopping, maybe for groceries and other times for clothes. Some times I would have to invent ideas. It just seemed that I could not keep him home early in the day. We would also go for lunch; usually it was a late lunch early dinner.

Sometimes when we were out Jim would get separated from me, be it at the grocery store or a restaurant. Jim couldn't seem to find me easily. One time at the store I was checking out and Jim had to go to the bathroom. I thought he would be okay. The restrooms were directly across from the checkout line. I was only about two people back from the cashier, but too much time had gone by. Jim should have been back, but by the time he came out of the restroom he was lost. I finally spotted him pacing up and down in front of the checkouts looking lost. I got his attention and the normal reaction from him was anger. After that I started wearing very brightly colored clothes; almost neon colors. I wanted to make sure if that situation arose again he would be able to spot me. It did help a lot but from then on when we were out like that I always made sure I was right outside the restroom waiting for him. By late afternoon Jim would be ready to come home. He did not want to be out when it started to get dark.

I realized that, when on one occasion we were at a relative's house and had to drive home in the dark. Jim was very upset. I kept telling him I was being careful. I couldn't go very fast, not that I was over the speed limit, but Jim was paranoid about the speed and thought I was going too fast. When we finally did get home it took a while for him to settle down.

At the time I did not know that those episodes were part of sun downing. Wherever we went after that I made sure we were home before dark. As the cold months started coming in at the end of 2005, Jim hated the cold and little by little we stayed in the house. Eventually, he did not want to go anywhere.

When I did have to get Jim out for a doctor's appointment, I would have to start getting him ready a good two hours before it was time to leave. At first he could pretty much shower by himself. I would help him into the tub and Jim could get his shower. As time went on, I had to get the water going for him, make sure it wasn't too hot and warn him when I would actually turn the shower on. If I didn't do that Jim would get really upset. I had to be very gentle with him just like you would with a child first learning to be in the shower.

I had to make sure that he didn't feel rushed. That was another bone of contention. Jim would get mad if he thought I was rushing him. Once showering was done, dressing became the next issue. At first he only had trouble with his belt. Then the rest of his clothes became troublesome for him to put on. Jim once came to me and asked if his jeans were on backwards. Well they were. He knew something was wrong with his clothes but couldn't figure it out.

At last with all the confrontations that were going on, I finally learned not to yell or make any snide remarks. I would just gently guide him back to the bedroom and get his jeans on the right way. It became apparent rather quickly that Jim could no longer dress himself without it being a total disaster. I had to dress him myself from his underwear to his outerwear, trying to do it without getting him upset because he couldn't do it himself. It was a chore that became very exasperating. I got the knack but it took quite a while. It wasn't always easy.

We always had eaten our dinners on snack trays in the living room while watching television. We had done this since the day we were married. There were a lot of times when Jim got frustrated or mad at dinner time. He had lots of complaints. Each time was always different. Sometimes Jim would refuse to eat, making some kind of excuse. Maybe I said something wrong not knowing I said it wrong, or in the wrong manner. Jim seemed to get a different meaning out of the words spoken. I now know that because of the symptoms of Alzheimer's, Jim's brain would not allow him to process the words correctly so his response was altogether different than what I had expected.

Usually it was anger. Because of this I started dreading dinner time. It mostly ended in a disaster.

When Jim really was upset at dinner, food would go flying all over the carpet. He liked to have wine with dinner too. You can imagine the mess. Spaghetti sauce and red wine all over a light colored carpet. I don't know how many times the carpet was cleaned in that period of time. I was at my wits end. There was so much yelling and screaming. I know that I shouldn't have yelled, but when some one is yelling and screaming at you the natural instinct is to yell back. Jim was probably totally confused about what was happening. It was the disease, not him.

Some where in there I got the bright idea to get a new dinning room table. The one we had was like a picnic table with benches. This did not lend to a nice dinner for two. It worked well for company, but that was about all. We bought a round table with regular chairs. It was working out very nicely. Dinner started to be more pleasing.

I bought a round flannel backed table clothes with elastic around the edge. This kept it fitted to the table and there were not any more spills because of a loose table cloth.

As the dinners seemed to be going much smoother, Jim was having trouble with finding the silverware and being able to put his drinking glass down without spilling. I starting watching and soon realized that Jim's depth perception and ability to distinguish colors was not there. The original table cloth I bought was grey to match with the carpet. I had to put aside the notion of trying to make things look pretty and make them functional.

I bought a green table cloth to help contrast with the silverware. Then I started giving Jim a red glass to drink from. I also started using different color plates. If I made light colored food I would use the brown stoneware and if I made dark colored food I would use the white corelle ware. That sure made dinners a lot easier.

Soon, Jim was starting to have more problems. He was depressed and having a hard time sleeping. When he got like this and we would have some of our evening conversations he would be upset over the whole situation and tell me to just "shoot me". Another phase he would use was "they shoot horses don't they"? It seemed to me that at these times Jim was well aware of all the things going wrong with him.

Jim didn't talk too much of his AD, but I think deep down inside he knew what the outcome would be.

The drugs that Jim was taking didn't seem to be working the way they were suppose to. We were on a regular schedule of doctor visits to his neurologist, who was trying new and different drugs. All the side effects that were bad were the ones Jim would have. I kept track by using WEBMD™ as my guide.

Jim was also given Adivan, which is a sedative similar to Valium, but not as strong. So I am told. This drug was also causing more agitation, but it was prescribed after one of his trips to the ER. The Adivan seemed to becoming addictive because the time between Jim's doses was getting shorter and shorter.

Some times Jim would bulk at the fact that he was taking so many drugs. Some of his medications were switched to liquid because he was starting to have a hard time swallowing. Not all of the drugs could be switched, but the ones that were could be mixed with another liquid to make it easier to go down. One night I was giving Jim one of his medicines and I asked him to drink the water. He got part of it down. I said there was some left and he needed to drink it. Well, Jim just turned the glass upside down and poured it on the floor and said "there it's down". Things were going down hill with the medicines. I had a hard time getting him quieted down in the evening. That was when he was to take the Adivan. Because he would drink wine I finally decided that was the only way to get the drugs in him. I would crush the pills and mix them into the wine. He drank it and off to sleep he went.

On one particular trip to the ER, I called the ambulance. Jim was highly agitated and I did not want to drive him myself. There were other times like this when I did drive and Jim would lash out at me while I was driving. I didn't want to take that chance again. This time the doctor admitted Jim into to the hospital for further observation. It lasted for about five days. I stayed with Jim the whole time, even overnight. The doctors wanted Jim to go into the psychiatric ward so they could watch how he would react to a change in medications. They explained that I would not be allowed to stay with him; I am not sure even if there were any kind of visiting hours. If Jim would not sign papers to go voluntarily then the doctors wanted me to commit him. Jim and I both started to cry. There was no way I could do that to him.

After talking with the doctors and trying to work out a plan to help Jim they finally let him come home. I had to sign papers to agree to their terms. One was to stop Jim from drinking. I knew I had a long road to haul. I felt I could handle that in due time.

It was after this hospital stay that Jim started seeing a psychiatrist on a regular basis. It was the best thing that had happened. Every thing seemed to mellow out for a while. Little by little Jim stopped drinking wine. I think mostly in part because he could no longer hold the glass. I would have to pick it up and put it down for him or else he would spill it. Then it progressed to where I would have to hold the glass while he drank from it. It took a while for this to happen but eventually he quit asking for a glass of wine.

It was around this time that Jim was having trouble holding onto his silverware when eating. I had to start feeding him. It was a slow process. Jim still wanted to be able to do it himself, but it just did not work. I also had to walk him to the dinner table and tell him where he was to sit. Jim could not remember.

We were staying at home more and more. Jim didn't want to go out anywhere. Most of the time I couldn't even get him to go on the porch to sit. Our back porch is a little high - one story. But then I remembered our trip to Florida and how he didn't want to be on the balcony. I would try to take Jim's arm and walk out onto the porch. He would go with me but it was only for a minute or so. I would then have to take him back into the house.

I was having trouble taking him to the grocery store too. I would try to get him to sit in the car. He would be so stiff. I had to place him in the seat and put his legs in one at a time. There were times when Jim would try to sit backwards in the passenger seat. I had a hard time trying to get him turned to sit the right way. When I did get Jim out for some shopping, we could never go far. If he had to go to the bathroom Jim wouldn't go in a public restroom. He said something to the effect that it was too open. Needless to say we stopped shopping.

Jim couldn't always find the bathroom at home. I would take him by the hand and walk him down the hall. Jim would have to sit. He always missed whenever he would stand. The few times that Jim would attempt to use the bathroom by himself, he would come to me afterwards and explain that the seat was wet but didn't know how it got that way. That was a fiasco. Jim would argue with me about it. I tried to explain but again his reasoning powers were being lost.

When I first stopped taking Jim grocery shopping it was okay. I made sure of what I needed and get in and out of the store quickly so I would only be gone an hour. But I had to stop doing that. We needed bread and milk one day. I told Jim I would only be gone ten minutes. I was only going to the convenience store down the hill. When I left he was quietly sitting on the sofa watching television and I figured ten minutes would be okay. By the time I did get back, which was less than ten minutes, Jim was pacing up and down the hall way looking for the bathroom. I made sure I kept all the lights on so he could see everything, but even that did not work.

2006

Jim was getting his days and nights mixed up. I wasn't getting any sleep. The tension was getting worse. He would be up roaming around wanting something to eat. One night at two a.m. he stood at the bottom of the bed demanding coffee. Jim said "I want my coffee and I want it now" in no uncertain terms. I got up made him coffee and before it was done Jim was asleep on the couch.

Some times when he was sitting in the living room he would call for me, asking me, "Where are you?" Or "Come and get me". At times when we sat together on the couch he at one end and me at the other, Jim seemed to be in a world of his own. He would be very quiet for a period of time and then ask me,"Where have you been, where did you go?". I would tell I was there all the time. Jim would say that he lost some time and did not know what happened.

One of the hardest things that went on was when Jim would ask to go home. At first I would tell him, "this is where you live" and "you are already home". He would fight and argue about it. I didn't know what to say. But as this going home question persisted I learned to avert it. I would tell him he was staying with me for the night. It would be okay for him to stay. The experts tell me that he probably was thinking of his home when he was a young boy. A lot of Alzheimer's patients say they want to go home.

I don't know if wandering is in connection with wanting to go home or not. Jim only had one episode with wandering. We had the deck re-stained after putting a roof on it. While it was drying Jim and I sat in the front yard on lawn chairs. It was a beautiful sunny, warm day. Jim just loved that kind of weather. It was one of his good days or so I thought. We got to talking about something that I can't remember now, but whatever it was, we went onto the computer to look. I think we were talking about buying something. I had left the lawn chairs outside and the front door open. It was just so pretty out and all the sun shine came in. It made everything look so cheery.

Jim sat with me for awhile at the computer. I explained everything I was doing. He either got bored or forgot what we were doing on the computer. Jim left the room and I quickly finished the transaction. It was only a matter of minutes.

I went to the living room, thinking he was watching the television. He wasn't there. I looked down stairs. He wasn't there. I thought to myself, he went back outside to sit. He wasn't there either.

My heart starting pounding not knowing where he had gone; never thought that he would walk away from the house. Just then the neighbor from across the street, who also is a very good friend, called over to me. He said Jim had just walked down the street. I never even bothered to put my shoes on.

The two of us went after Jim. As we got to the corner a lady driving up the connecting road slowed down to ask if we were looking for a man walking. She said he was down the road and looked really confused. The neighbor and I picked up the pace to a run. Jim had gotten what was about three blocks. He was more to the center of the road than to the side. At that time of day most people were coming home from work, so it was pretty busy. Jim was walking in a circle scratching his head. That was usually the sign when he had no idea where he was or what he was doing. I was careful not to yell and scare him. I tried to be jovial asking if he was out for a walk. Jim sort of answered me with a yes but I could see that he was upset. I gently took his arm in mine, turned him around and headed back to the house.

The neighbor followed suit trying to keep the situation on a light note. Jim and I talked to the neighbor for a short time trying to keep normal. I finally got Jim back in the house settled him on the sofa. I made sure the television was on and hoped it would keep Jim's attention for a few minutes. I quickly brought the lawn chairs in closed and locked the front door. I did not want Jim to wander out again. That was the only and the last time I let the front door open. It could have been tragic, thankfully it was not.

It was all so heart breaking. Jim looked like a little lost puppy. All I wanted to do was put my arms around him and hug him. But sometimes the confusion of the disease wouldn't let me do that.

It was getting harder to handle Jim. I couldn't leave the house with him or without him. The frustration for both Jim and I was too great to handle. I started to hate more than love. I knew it was getting time to get help. I didn't know which way to turn.

Luckily my sister-in-law is good friends with the director of one of the Alzheimer's assisted living care homes. I made an appointment with her about a year or so before all of this started to happen. We talked for a good three hours and she gave me a tour of the home. I was very impressed and knew when the time came that this was were I would have Jim live. That time came. I knew it was coming. But it was so hard to do.

Our nephew, who is a psychiatrist and did his PHD studies in family diseases, one of which he did research into Alzheimer's disease, knew before I did that it was time for Jim to go to a home. Our nephew had let me know that there would be a time that I could no longer care for Jim at home. He talked to me a lot, told me that because Jim had early onset AD that it would hit hard and fast. As time went on after Jim was in the home, I knew what our nephew was trying to tell me. He was concerned about this for my health too. Our nephew and Jim's brother both told me I had kept Jim home much too long. Jim needed more help than I could do by myself.

In the beginning of May 2006, the annual registration for the car came due. It was in both of our names. I had to get Jim to sign. Whenever I needed Jim to put his signature on any kind of papers, I made sure the table was clear, had a chair ready and the paper and pen right there on the table and the lights on bright so he could see everything. Up until this time he did okay with signing papers. I could read it pretty well. Never had anything come back to re-sign. This time was different. Jim could barely hold the pen. I can't remember if he did sign it or not but we always made sure we had duplicate registrations.

I knew right then and there I needed to get Power of Attorney (POA). We were getting ready to go to the grocery store. On the way is a notary. I was trying to figure out how to do this. I got Jim into the shower hoping that he would take a long shower. I hopped onto the computer and searched for a site for a POA. I found one almost immediately and looked it over. It seemed to fit the bill, although I no idea what I really needed. It only cost $20. I paid for it, downloaded and did a printout, all in of a matter of ten minutes. I couldn't believe how quick it all happened. It was a good thing. Jim must have taken one of the shortest showers on record. After I had gotten him dressed and about ready to leave, I sat down on the sofa with Jim and gave him a very short explanation of the papers. I told him it would allow me to take care of all the finances. He said okay and we were on our way.

I explained the situation to the notary and we began to sign the papers. I had a tough time getting Jim to even see the paper let alone sign them. He had the two main pages signed but because we couldn't really read Jim's signature, the notary put her initials and signature beside his. Then we started through the pages. Jim had to initial each page. There are seventeen pages to this document. I just looked at the notary and shrugged my shoulders. She said he had to initial the pages which meant that he read it and knew what he was signing. Jim was standing there rather quiet as if he didn't know what was going on. Next thing I knew he looked up and said to the notary "She is going to get everything anyway". That was all she needed to hear. She put her stamp on it and off we went.

The POA was a godsend. Within three weeks from then he would be in a home. It was about a week before Jim went to the home that everything started to fall apart. I couldn't keep Jim happy no matter what I did. I couldn't sleep and I couldn't get anything done. All we did was sit on the couch and watch television. I was in contact with the director of the home. I had to communicate with her over the fax machine. It was in the back bedroom. I kept the door closed so he could not hear it. I couldn't talk to her on the phone. I didn't want Jim to hear what I was saying. She was going to send me papers to sign which she could hold for thirty days. I figured I could work something out in thirty days.

That was over a Friday and Saturday that I faxed the Director all that was going on. On Monday morning about 6 am, Jim and I were trying to have our morning coffee. As I was fixing it, Jim said to me so clear and straight forward that I couldn't believe my ears. He said "you know I have Alzheimer's and I need help. I need to be in the hospital". All I could say was I will take care of it. He was very quiet that morning. I finished making coffee and we sat for a while. About 8 am Jim said

"Nobody is listening and I need help". I told him I would call the doctor. I called the director and told her what had happened. She told me "Do it now".

The decision was taken out of my hands. Jim had asked for help. I had to take him to the hospital for a 23 hour observation. Needless to say some of the doctors are NOT educated in Alzheimer's patients. To me it seemed like they were asking stupid questions.

Later I found out that those kinds of questions were in a way an evaluation. I talked and talked to a social worker and explained almost word for word what the director said should be done. Jim had to have some tests done. One of them was a brain scan. I was with him almost all the way. When we got to the x-ray unit for the brain scan the technician was asking me questions. She asked if it was from a fall. I explained that he was going to an assisted living home and needed these test done. She turned to me and asked if this was a formality. I said yes and she understood the rest.

If it wasn't for the director of the home I would never have gotten through the process. She walked me through everything. I can't thank her enough for all she did. She is just wonderful. It seemed like I was on the phone constantly with her. I had no idea what all I was supposed to do. She told me once Jim was settled in the hospital room for the night to go home. She told me do not spend the night. It was too stressful. I called Jim's brothers to let them know. I must have talked for hours with them. I then called my sister and my two brothers and talked to them for hours. To say the least it was not a good nights' sleep. Everyone was very supportive. I had always tried to keep everyone up-to-date with Jim's behavior. Everyone else knew it was time for more extensive care for Jim way before I knew it.

The next morning came too early. I got a call from the hospital asking me when some one from the family would be there. I asked if there was a problem and they said not really. Jim was just walking around following the nurses and they didn't know what to do with him. I explained that he was to go to the assisted living home and that an ambulance would be there to get him.

Again I called the director, told her about the call. She told me just to come to the home and Jim would be there around eleven. She was on the phone taking care of all the details knowing exactly what should be done.

I got to the home and waited in their conference room. I could see outside and watch for the ambulance. The whole time I was fighting back tears. It was on of those moments in your life that you never forget. The director told me that Jim would not be able to see me, but I just couldn't stand at the window and watch. I stood back against the wall. I could see him. Jim looked like a little boy looking around at something new. He was very calm. He had his head up trying to see things, but I am only guessing. He looked like a turtle sticking his head out of his shell. As I look back, Jim was so very innocent looking, but at the time it was the most devastating time of my life. I had many decisions to make and papers to sign. After that was done I knew Jim would never be coming home again.

That first day at the home was extremely hard. My emotions were like a rollercoaster. I knew that Jim needed the kind of care I just couldn't provide – 24 hrs. Now it didn't matter if he was up all night roaming around. The caregivers were always there along with nurses and other staff to help.

I had a hard time just going into the living area of the home. The director had to keep encouraging me that it would be alright. She was excellent at her job. She just kept talking to me saying to think of the home and the people as an extended family. I would make friends with the other family members and we could share our stories; console each other by just talking everything over. This is exactly what eventually happened. The director told me not to think of it as putting Jim away.

She finally got me back to where Jim was. I only peeked around the corner to see how he was doing. I felt very timid about going to him.

It was lunchtime. Jim was sitting at the table getting ready to eat. He still had on the hospital gown. I got the courage to go to him. I put my arms around him and just held him for awhile; giving him lots of kisses. I reassured Jim that it was all okay. He would be well taken care of. At that point I realized that he had no underwear on under the gown. I was so upset that the hospital nurses hadn't taken care of Jim. He is such a private, modest person when it came to things like that. It was so indignant on the part of the hospital. I was just so upset. Jim would not have been happy at all if he understood. Sometimes the hospital staff has no clue how to handle an Alzheimer's patient.

Immediately after lunch Jim was taken to get a shower and was dressed in clean clothes. It had been about two or three days since he had a shower. The caregivers took over right away, putting all of their skills to work. They were so calm and soothing, and put Jim at ease. Of course he looked to me with a question on his face. I told Jim it was okay. Everything would be fine.

While Jim was in the shower I had a chance to talk to the caregivers. Being brand new to the home the caregivers did not know who I was. When I started talking to them about

Jim I could see quizzical looks from them. They kept looking back and forth to each other. I then realized I was wearing the same colors they were, navy blue top and khaki pants. That is their uniform but with a casual look. They thought they were talking to a newly hired caregiver, wondering why I had tears in my eyes. They were trying to tell me that there were no tears in there. The caregivers do their best only to be happy. I did not have a visitors tag on my shirt so they were a bit confused. Once I explained who I was they put their arms around me to give me a hug. There was only one other time I wore those colors. When some of the other residents started to look to me for help I knew I couldn't wear that outfit again. The caregivers understood, calming all of my fears. I told them some things to look for with handling Jim. How he reacted to different situations that I had been through with him. I explained that Jim had been treated with kid gloves and he was spoiled. The fact that we never had children lended to the fact that I catered to almost every whim. Jim usually got whatever he wanted.

After Jim's shower we went to his room. The director was sitting in the chair putting Jim's name on all his clothes. I told her I would do that but she said to take Jim out and walk around the building and get familiar with the area.

Jim and I walked around looking at everything. The building has four wings called houses. They each have a different paint scheme which helps the residents identify their house. In the center is a big square that has several rooms. We could walk around in a big circle. They have a big community room where the daily activities are held and a very large long kitchen for morning coffee, get-to-gethers and reading the morning paper. Off to the sides of this big hallway are alcoves that have settees and chairs for alternative visiting areas. As Jim and I walked seeing all of this, he would tell me how pretty everything looked. He actually used the word beautiful.

Jim kept asking me what this place is and why was he here. I had a hold of his arm the whole time we were walking. I would pat Jim's hand, reassure him that he was here for rehabilitation and therapy, and for the help he had asked for. Jim said okay, and just kept saying how beautiful everything looked. I had to keep telling him that they would take good care of him. I kept reiterating that the professionals were here to help. Jim sort of smiled and seemed to understand.

The nurses at the home needed to check Jim over, blood pressure, heart rate, temperature. They even took his picture to put in the daily log book for recognition purposes because he was new. As they were doing that I had some time to talk to the director. I didn't know how I would handle leaving when the time came. She told me not to over think what actions I might take. She said to try to be easy on myself. The director said the caregivers would provide a diversion, take Jim's attention away from me so I could slip out. She thought the best thing to do was not say the words "good-bye". It would be a signal that I wasn't going to be there. It might make Jim upset. She said as time went on I would find ways to leave without him thinking I was leaving which I eventually did.

That first day it was getting time for me to go home. I was fretting about it. Not really knowing how I was going to do this even though the director had given me advice on what to do. It was dinner time and the caregiver came to Jim, took him by the hands and led him into the dinner room. It was the perfect diversion. I slowly backed away. The caregiver could see me out of the corner of her eye. She knew. She just nodded her head and I quietly left. That was the worst day in my life. I was going home to an empty house, not sure of how I was going to cope with Jim not being there.

When I got home I had a dozen or so phone calls to make to all the family. I had three phones going, two cells and one home. As the batteries wore out I changed to a different phone. Finally all was said and done. I was totally exhausted, physically, mentally and emotionally. I don't remember how well I slept that night. It was totally quiet and empty without Jim being there.

The second day I got to the home around lunchtime. Jim was already seated at the dinning room table. Again I approached him very tentatively, trying to brace myself for any reactions. I went to him; put my arms around him, giving him a hug and a kiss. I did my best not to say a big "HI" trying not to signal him that I was really away. Next thing I saw were tears rolling down his face. It was all I could do not to cry myself. The director warned me that AD patients are very sensitive to emotions, like the look on my face and tension in my body. I had to be very careful.

I took my hanky and wiped away Jim's tears. He asked me not to leave him alone again. This just reinforced the fact I needed to portray that I was always there. I think I told him I was doing the wash and putting away clothes. It seemed to make Jim feel better. I helped him finish eating his lunch. I made sure from that day on he felt that I was only in the other room doing housework. I used the same phrases that I would have if he were home. I tell him I will be down the hall as if going to the bathroom or going to the bedroom to get something for him or putting laundry away. I tell him that I will be in the kitchen fixing lunch or putting away dishes. As long as I can give Jim an explanation as to what I am doing he seems to be okay with that.

It is very hard but I have learned to put my emotions on hold when I visit. I cannot let Jim see me cry or let him sense I am upset. There have been days when I had to leave earlier than I wanted. In those first months after Jim went into the home there were a lot of ups and downs.

When Jim would get upset because he couldn't say or do anything that his brain would not let him, his reactions were not always appropriate. I didn't know how to handle this and my reaction was and still is to cry. One day it was really bad. I hid my face from Jim and I said something to the effect that I had to get something from the bedroom and would be back in a few minutes. I left in tears. I tried to talk to the director but it seemed that all I was doing was crying. I told her I thought I should go home. She was very concerned too and agreed. After that if I was having a bad day I most likely did not visit Jim. This may sound a little crass but it really is the best way to handle that situation.

2007

I have been going to a psychologist to help me get through all of this. She has explained to me that those feelings are all okay. I have to keep living too. I have all the finances to take care of along with keeping up the house and all the other work entailed with daily living. This will happen. She has encouraged me to take at least one day to do things for myself. So as time goes on I do take a day a week and call it my "at home day". I take some time for myself and also get things done around the house. The next day when I go to see Jim I feel much better and more refreshed. I am able to handle his situation better.

I have a great support system with all of my family and Jim's family. They have all given me great guidance and understanding. They back me up on all the decisions that I have made and told me that whatever I think is best for Jim is fine with them. I have seen where other family members from the home have had a very bad time with their family members not understanding all the decisions and all the heartache that goes with having a spouse with Alzheimer's disease. I am so grateful for the love all my family and friends have given me.

I also have a very dear girl friend. We have been friends for almost forty years. I can tell her everything and anything. She never passes judgment, but gives me ideas on how to handle different things. I feel so much better after I have talked to her. I can be mad, I can be crying, and she is always there for me.

As time goes on I have learned to stay calm. I sit back and watch taking in how other residents react to different comments or conversations. It gives me some insight on how to handle everyday living with Alzheimer's. I have learned that I cannot always answer questions for Jim or for others. I have to go into their world. What ever is happening now for me is not the same for Jim either. One day he asked me what school he was in. I told him West Mifflin. This is where we went to high school together. Most of the time a simple answer is the best. If I try to go into a deeper explanation and Jim has a puzzled look on his face, I know I went too far with trying to answer him.

Basically all that I can do is to cajole and redirect, go along with what ever Jim is saying. He usually only hears the last word that I have said to him. One day I was walking him to lunch. Jim asked where we were going. I told him we were headed into the dining room to sit. All he heard was the word sit. Jim started to sit down right where we were standing and almost ended on the floor. That is when I realized I could only tell him one thing at a time.

I have learned from the caregivers what to do and what not to do. I usually follow suit with the same terminology that they use. I think it helps to have some continuity. Jim doesn't seem to be mixed up when trying to get him to do anything. One particular thing is when Jim is eating. The caregivers almost always use the term "big bite" when it is dinner time. It is the easiest way to get Jim or the other residents to open their mouths. Most of the time, he seems to sense the food is ready for him. He automatically will open his mouth for the next bite. He looks like a little bird at feeding time.

There are many times when I just step back and let the caregivers take over. Sometimes there are too many people around and Jim gets even more confused. He doesn't like sudden movements or loud noises.

With so much going on it is best for me to move out of the way. Jim needs to be handled gently. When I talk to him I try not to be too loud and explain what I am doing as I go along. I would tell him that I was buttoning his shirt or straitening his pants, or pulling up his socks. I would say to Jim, "that should be more comfortable". He would look up at me and give me a big smile.

There was one time I had to step in and take over. I came in one day found Jim in his bedroom only half dressed. He was walking in circles scratching his head. This was always a sign that he was more than just confused. Jim had his shirt and pants on but he had no diaper on. Not knowing what had transpired I finished dressing him. I explained everything I was doing. I put on his diaper pulled up his pants, and buttoned his shirt. I had to get him dry socks. I got those on and then put on his slippers. I stood him up and pulled up his pants. I then realized the pants were on backwards. I was not about to undress him just to get his pants on front wards.

It didn't matter because he has knit pants that have an elastic waist and no one would know the difference anyway. It all looked the same so I let it go. By this time Jim had calmed down but I think at this point he thought I was one of the caregivers. I was okay with that. I took Jim into the living room and sat him in his chair. Everything was alright. But then I saw the caregiver in the kitchen doing dishes and wondered why Jim was left like that in his bedroom. The nurse then came by and told me Jim had socked the caregiver a good one in the jaw. I felt terrible about it and went to talk to her and apologized for Jim. She told me if it wasn't for the disease she would have hit him back. I was stunned at her comment. It just didn't sit right with me. After that I started watching her to see how she handled other residents. From her actions I could see she was just doing a JOB. She just wanted to put her time in and get a paycheck.

There was one more incident that Jim hit this same caregiver in the chest. When I found out about it I went to the director and re-itinerated about Jim having a stubborn streak. If he wasn't ready to do something he would not do it. All he needed was a little space. Then the caregiver could give it a little time and start over, but this time talk Jim through everything and take it a little slower. That is why he hit her. Jim did not know what was going on. She did not want to take the time to "care" for him. Needless to say it wasn't long after that the caregiver was let go.

With talking this over with the director, she explained that some of the girls know after a week or so that they are not cut out to do this kind of work and would quit on their own without having to be fired. The director keeps a really good finger on this kind of behavior.

The caregivers that are now in Jim's house are just spectacular, I can't say enough of the wonderful job they do, not only for Jim but they take care of me too. When they see that I am upset, we talk, we cry, and they always have a hug for me. They try to console me with their words of wisdom. Many of them have had AD in their family too.

Everyday when I come in and when I am ready to leave; there are always hugs and kisses for each of them. They always reassure me that Jim is well taken care of. That means so much. It is hard enough leaving Jim and the caregivers always soothe it over.

One of the things I was always told is to try to keep a sense of humor. Look for the funny things. Some people would be upset thinking that I or other family members were laughing at the residents, but they can be so comical at times you really do have to laugh.

There was one gentleman who was there everyday visiting his wife, who has since had to move on to skilled nursing. He knows Jim's side of the family and was more familiar with us. He would always call to Jim using Jim's full name. Most of the time Jim would smile and say hi, but this one particular day Jim seemed to be ignoring the man. Well he called out to Jim and Jim did not answer. The man called out to Jim again. It took a few seconds. Jim turned a little in this man's direction and called him "asshole". Everybody laughed and the man did not seem to be upset. It only goes to show that the gears are working, just that it may take time for the words. That story has been told and retold and every one gets a chuckle out of it.

On occasion the caregivers will bring their kids if they can't get a baby sitter. There was this little girl, maybe a year or so old and the residents were enjoying watching her run around and playing. The little girl came over to Jim's chair. She was giggling, waved her little hand and saying hello to Jim. He looked up to see her and the next thing he said was "they sure are making them small these days". Well you should have heard the laughter. It made the atmosphere for that day quite jovial.

On the other hand you have to be careful of what is said. Some of the residents can get quite upset if not handled well. There is one lady who always wants to get out. She is always asking when she can get out of here. The same gentleman that was always calling to Jim answered her but it was not good. She had kept saying she wanted out and he told her "you are locked in and can't get out'". He said this very loudly and rather nastily.

She was totally upset and I think it took some doing to get her calmed down. I was upset too. I don't talk like that to Jim and I try to give him the impression that he is not "locked up" in a home. I went over to this man and quietly told him that he couldn't say things like that. It is too upsetting for her and other residents. I don't know if the man got the gist of what I was trying to tell him but after that he never said anything to her like that again. I was glad. There are just certain things that can't be said. I make sure I weigh my words before speaking.

There are many sad incidents but one in particular, which I just recently found out about. One of the male residents seemed to be doing pretty well. He was quiet and seemed to be a gentle soul. For whatever reason, he had gone to the hospital and never returned. I asked about him. I guess that when he had come to the home he had not been told he had AD. While he was in the hospital some one told him, the man just gave up and not long after that he passed away. He just did not want to live anymore. It is just so sad.

Jim's one year anniversary recently passed, May 16, 2007. I think he is coming into the last stage of AD. He was 180lbs at this time last year and he is now 133 lbs. I was told that this can be a wasting disease and could happen to Jim. It is hard to say what stage he is in because of all the crossovers between stages.

Things seem to be a lot calmer than when he first went to the home. He was doing a lot of walking, but he would lose his balance very easily. Jim would not know to put his hands in front of himself to break a fall. Once he slid off the couch and hit face first. He spent the day in the hospital. They had thought that he may have broken his nose. Thankfully it was not, but there were two black eyes. Once he had staples in the back of his head and then most recently he had ten stitches in his forehead. The falls just happen so quickly and then it seems to go in slow motion. It is nobody's fault. It is part of the disease.

Hospice was called in between Christmas and New Years. Jim has had a lot more care with the help of the hospice aides and the nurses. He does very little walking and when he does the caregivers are beside him. Jim tires very easily too. Once he has had his shower in the mornings and then breakfast he may walk a bit. But it doesn't take long and he is in his chair and napping. Some of the medicine Jim gets is to help keep him calmed down. I gave them permission to do so. With all the falls he took and many bumps on the head, some which did not required a hospital visit, but none the less gave him many bruises. There was one fall that cracked a bone in his shoulder. We didn't know that for a little while, he was getting Tylenol and ibuprofen which helped but I could tell that Jim was hurting. The mobile unit for x-rays came in and found the crack. They tried to get him to wear a sling, but Jim kept taking it off. It took awhile but it finally healed.

Jim has a hospital bed that can be lowered and not have the fear of him falling out of bed. There is a pad that is put on the floor next to his bed as a precaution in case he would roll out of bed.

He has been using a wheelchair. There is a lot of time when the caregivers or the hospice aide can not get Jim to stand. Hospice provided the chair a few weeks ago.

Jim sleeps a lot more now. As I said before the morning activities just zaps his energy. He is usually asleep by the time I get there. Sometimes I have trouble waking him for lunch and more times than not, he does not wake up until later. The caregivers then feed him, give him his medicine and then take him to the bathroom. By then he is exhausted again and Jim will nap pretty much the rest of the afternoon.

Dinner is served around 5pm and then it is the same routine after dinner. I have been there at those times and Jim is asleep.

I have talked to the caregivers on the evening shift 3-11. They have told me when Jim does start to fall asleep in his chair the will put him to bed. It is usually around 7:30 or so. He is up at 6am; for Jim that is now a long day.

When Jim is awake when I first go in, I talk to him about the weather, maybe I will talk about the Steelers or the Pirates. I try to find small bits and pieces that I think he may understand. Sometimes a small smile will come across his face.

I try to get Jim to smile. Always telling him how nice his smile is and ask him to show me his pearly whites. It works most of the time. I tell him how nice he looks, using the word spiffy and how nice his hair look, even if it is standing straight up in the air. Jim seems to like that.

It's hard to hug him because he is always sitting. I give him kisses all the time and tell him "I love you". Most of the time his eyes are closed and I am not sure if he hears me but at other times I do get a reaction of some kind.

I hold his hand, pat it and kiss it. One day recently I was doing just that. Jim took my hand. At first I thought he was upset about something and was going to squeeze my hand really hard. He has done that before when he was frustrated. I just never know.

Jim's eyes were closed. He gently took my hand and put it to his lips and gave me a soft gentle kiss. The tears just flowed down my face. I was so glad his eyes were closed. I did not want him to see me cry.

I feel this was his way of saying I love you too, even though it took him a while to do so.

So far no more falls. He does get riled up in the morning when the hospice aide is there. He has hit her and spit at her and gives her a bad time when she tries to give him his shower. Afterwards he does settle down. It has to be a trying time for Jim, having someone bathing him. The caregivers understand and try to give him as much space as they can. The caregivers have starting giving Jim his medicine about an hour before the aide comes. It helps.

I have talked with the hospice nurse about some of the drugs Jim has been taking. She and I decided that is would be okay to take him off his high blood pressure and cholesterol medicine. With his weight so low there should not be any affect. We also talked over about taking him off Aricept. Aricept is good for in the early stages of Alzheimer's. Jim has been on it for 5 years. We felt that it was really not doing anything for him. They give him medicine to keep him calm, which we talked to great lengths about.

I told them I would rather see him calm then trying to walk all over the place and be afraid of him falling and hurting himself. I don't want to see him in the hospital anymore with black eyes, bruises or stitches in his forehead. It hurts too much.

I have to wait to see what the future holds. It is not good or maybe it would be a blessing. Jim has to know somewhere in the back of his mind that he is not at home and other people have to care for him. I don't think, if he really knew, that he would want it this way. I just hope he understands. I don't want him to hate me. I have a fear of that. I love Jim so much.

I have already lost Jimmy; most of the time I don't think he knows who I am. I tell him my name and he gives me a big smile. God has His reasons for how our lives turn out. I think He has given me strength to do what I have to.

I started volunteering; helping where I can with fund raising. I feel that in someway this is helping Jim. I needed to do something to help him out and I feel that this will keep me strong for Jim's sake.

In many of our conversations at home, Jim told me he did not want to be forgotten. I hope by telling the story of Jim's Journey that I have been able to keep that from happening.

With my heart on my sleeve, when it is Jim's time I will have lost the love of my life.

My brother wrote an article for H.O.G. TALES™ which I feel also needs to be included in "Jim's Journey" As the book goes to press the article has not been published in the magazine.

Zed gave me permission to use his story.

Jim's FXR

By Zed Kalbaugh

Jim has been part of my life longer than any one person outside of my parents and siblings. Jim and my sister, Gretchen, started dating when I was 6 years old. When Jim and Gretchen married I had more than a brother-in-law, I had a friend, confidant, and mentor. Jim became my big brother.

Jim and Gretchen included me in a lot of their life when I was a youngster. I loved to tag along with Jim to help with anything he might be doing. One of my favorite memories was going to local stock car races with them on Saturday night. Jim's interest turned to motorcycles before I was a teenager. He rode hare scrambles and cross country off road events on a street/trail Enduro. Later he rode a competition motocross bike. Finally he began to ride street bikes. I watched Jim as he worked on his bikes in my Dad's garage. He would tirelessly answer questions, telling me about two strokes, four strokes, pistons, cams, and valves. My interest in things mechanical took root. And then at last Jim gave me my first motorcycle ride. I had a tight grip around Jim and my grin filled his mirror. The hook had been set.

In later years, when I was home on leave from the Air Force Jim would lend me his motorcycle and I would take my future wife on dates. When I returned it to him after two weeks of riding with a fresh wash and wax, lubed chain, and filled gas tank he would say "I can't wait for you to borrow it again!"

I continued to actively ride street bikes but no Harley for me yet. A lot was happening in my life: marriage, school, and jobs for both my wife and me. Soon we had two beautiful children and were living in a different state than Jim. Fittingly, Jim's 1979 FXE Superglide was the first Harley I ever rode. I loved the sound and feel of it. He had just bought a new 1992 FXR Superglide we were riding together. I felt my next bike needed to be a Harley-Davidson. I found a 1992 Sportster with only 2900 miles on it and bought it in January 1993. The Sportster is a very capable motorcycle and I now have 80,000 miles on it.

MY sister, Gretchen wanted to ride, too, so she took a MSF rider class. She spent a season riding a 350cc street bike and the 1979 FXE. The next year she bought a new 1993 Sportster. The three of us got a chance to ride together that summer... all of us on Harleys.

Jim was quite an accomplished mechanic and he personally maintained every bike he ever owned. He also enjoyed doing his own customization and performance work. The 92 FXR was the perfect platform for him to create a personalized, high performance motorcycle. From the day Jim brought home the FXR it became a work in progress. Jim was very particular in making this bike a unique custom but not over done. He wanted it to be high performance but streetable, with instant torque and a broad powerband, while still running well on premium gasoline. What fantastic work he did! The list of modifications is long: Branch heads, roller rocker arms, performance camshaft, Super E carb with Thunderjet, K&N filter, tapered dual exhaust pipes, single fire high performance ignition with rev limiter, and an oil pressure gage to keep watch on it all. Jim also lowered the suspension front and rear with Progressive components, added custom wheels, a custom seat, a Harley-Davidson low rider custom tank and trim, and just the right amount of chrome. One of my favorite touches is some really cool chrome trim on the rear fender. This motorcycle is truly both show and go.

One day when we were out for a ride together, I was a bit taken aback when Jim offered to switch bikes so I could experience his pride and joy. After riding for awhile and taking it easy, try to get a feel for things. Jim pulled over to the side of the road and motioned me to come along side. He said "Listen, you need to find out what this bike it about. Go ahead and get on it! You are not going to hurt it". And so I did, within the bounds of the law, of course. The acceleration and torque were incredible. I had never ridden anything with such power and response. Little did I know that through a tremendous act of love and generosity some 10 years later this would be my next Harley-Davidson.

A few short years later Jim was diagnosed with early onset Alzheimer's disease. It has been heartbreaking to see the toll this terrible disease is having on Jim's life. I can only try to imagine the difficulty for my sister. Everyday routines became more and more difficult. Jim took an early retirement. His riding became less frequent and the distance shorter. For the first time in almost 40 years of owning and maintaining his own motorcycles this lifetime HOG member took his FXR to the local Harley dealer for service.

It pained me when he told me he wouldn't be riding anymore. He stayed with it as long as he could. I knew it had to hurt him badly. I told him "Jim, whenever I ride there is a part of you that rides with me". That brought a smile.

Eventually, a friend helped Jim and Gretchen get the bikes in condition to sell. Gretchen wasn't riding without Jim and the Sportster sold quickly. Jim would say that the FXR needed someone to ride it; both the thought of seeing it go was distressing to say the least. Jim and Gretchen discussed giving it away to make sure it got a good home and was appreciated for what it was and represented to both of them.

Gretchen sent me a hand written litter explaining all of this. Early that year Jim, at only 59 years of age, moved into an assisted living center because of the progression of his Alzheimer's disease. His motorcycle had not been run in well over a year. She was concerned that it would deteriorate. That motorcycle was made to be ridden and needed someone to take good care of it. Gretchen asked me to come and take it home. I was overwhelmed with emotion and I read her letter for the first time. I was going to be the one trusted with the care of Jim's beautiful Harley-Davidson.

Several months later I transported Jim's FXR from Pittsburgh to my home in Raleigh, NC. When I transferred the title I ordered a personalized license plate, JIMSFXR, to reflect my feeling that this will always be Jim's bike. I feel that I am a co-owner of sorts. Jim will always ride with me in spirit and I wanted his name on the bike. Jim launched me on this love affair with two wheels over 30 years ago and we continue to share in spirit.

An aircraft mechanic by trade, I do all my own motorcycle maintenance, the same way Jim did. I've need to make a few adjustments and tweak things a bit so that the bike will fit me, but I intend to keep it largely unchanged. Jim's customization and performance modifications will remain intake. It turns out the Jim's FXR and my XLH were both manufactured in October 1991. I refer to them as the twins and they keep each other company when they are parked for the night. I often get complemented on the FXR and I always tell the person that I can't take any credit for how great it is. Then I take the opportunity to tell a little bit about Jim.

Jim's battle with Alzheimer's continues but the disease is progressing. I hope that someday there will be a way to prevent it and ultimately a cure. If you have questions or concerns about Alzheimer's disease please visit alz.org. For now, I hope that Gretchen can take comfort in the knowledge that I will always take care of Jim's FXR and in that way Jim will be able to ride for as long as I do.

Jim lost his battle with Alzheimer's on February 19, 2008. I feel that I gave him the kind of funeral that he had asked for. I knew he wanted a church service. I had planned to have a service in the church we were married, but that church was shut down by the Catholic diocese. We had gone to a lot of services over the years at the Methodist church which my family had attended for years. Jim always liked that church. I had asked my sister-in-law, who is a Methodist Pastor if she would contact the minister and see if we could have the service there and if she would do the service. It all worked out very well.

I wanted to make sure he was remembered and honored with the things he was proudest, his military service in the Vietnam Era and his love of motorcycles. I invited the Patriot Guard and asked all of his friends who he rode with if they would also honor him with a motorcycle escort. My brother also brought JIMSFXR from Raleigh and led Jim's buddies in the procession.

Jim was buried in the National Cemetery of the Alleghenies with full military honors.

Jim is at peace now. There is no more worrying. Now I have to find my peace.

POSTSCRIPT

It is now January 2010; I had this book on the shelf long enough! I was having a difficult time every time I reread Jim's Journey, making sure I said what I wanted to say and that the spelling was all correct. It still brings tears to my eyes and I guess it always will.

I made friends with two great people just before Jim died; they gave me support and understanding in the months following Jim's death which gave me the strength I needed at the time. I will be forever grateful for the help they gave me.

I have moved on with my life as best I can. I kept waiting for things to return to normal, but they never did. Hospice sent me newsletters on what to expect through the grieving process. One of those things was that normal as I knew it will never be the same and I now had to find a new normal. I am not sure if I have found it yet, I am still working on that.

www.ingramcontent.com/pod-product-compliance
Lightning Source LLC
Chambersburg PA
CBHW060638290526
45793CB00001B/309